Jack and his Extra Y

Forward

The inspiration for the creation of this book comes from working with the families of children with X&Y chromosome variations both in the eXtraordinarY Kids Clinic and at family conferences around the world. There were so many times that we handed reading materials and textbook chapters to parents to learn more about their child's condition, while we had nothing to give their smart, curious children standing next to them. Also, parents often ask how to discuss the diagnosis with their child, but feel unprepared and ill-equipped to do so. This book was created to allow boys with XYY to learn more about their condition, and to facilitate the discussion between parents and their child about the diagnosis of XYY.

The author, Arlie Colvin, and the illustrator, Suzanne Hayes, have taken a complex topic and created a fantastic story that explains features of XYY in a way that kids will be able to understand. Jack's day captures the story of so many boys we see in the clinic--both children and parents will relate to his experiences. Truly understanding the diagnosis of XYY takes more than a diagram of chromosomes and can't be fully described by a medical textbook, and this book now provides that missing piece. We look forward to using this book as a tool to support boys with XYY and their families both today and in the years to come.

Nicole Tartaglia, MD

Susan Howell, MS, CGC

eXtraodinarY Kids Clinic
Children's Hospital Colorado
University of Colorado School of Medicine

Recommendations for using this resource.

Many parents of children with X&Y chromosome variations (also called sex chromosome aneuploidy or sex chromosome abnormalties) report feeling unprepared to talk with their child about the diagnosis. Most parents and adult individuals with X&Y chromosome variations say the discussion should happen early in life. It is our hope that this children's book can be used to introduce the topic to young children in an age-appropriate way. This book covers topics pertinent to children such as difficulties in school and visits to the doctor. In writing this story, we did not set out to mention every medical complication that may be experienced by individuals with this condition, but rather to address those which impact young children most.

- This book is intended for children with 47, XYY between the ages of 5 and 12 but can be read with individuals of any age.
- This is a story that a parent and child should read together.
- Talking about chromosomal variation is not a one-time event. Parents should expect to have many conversations with their child about this topic. This book can help with that discussion.
- Parents should invite their child to ask questions while reading this story. We hope that this story will encourage discussion between parent and child.
- We understand that not all boys with 47, XYY have the same experiences. For instance, not all children will require occupational therapy. It is at the discretion of the parents to decide which details to include or omit for their child.

Enjoy!

"Jaaaaack!" he hears his mom yell up the stairs. It's time to wake up for school. Sleepy, Jack says to his mother, "OK, OK, I'm coming." Jack sits up in bed, stretches and yawns. He has a big day ahead of him! As he stands up, he hears another voice in the hallway -- this time it's his sister. "Come on, Jack! You're going to make me late again!" Jack leaves his room and heads downstairs. "Leave me alone, Megan. I'm awake," he grumbles.

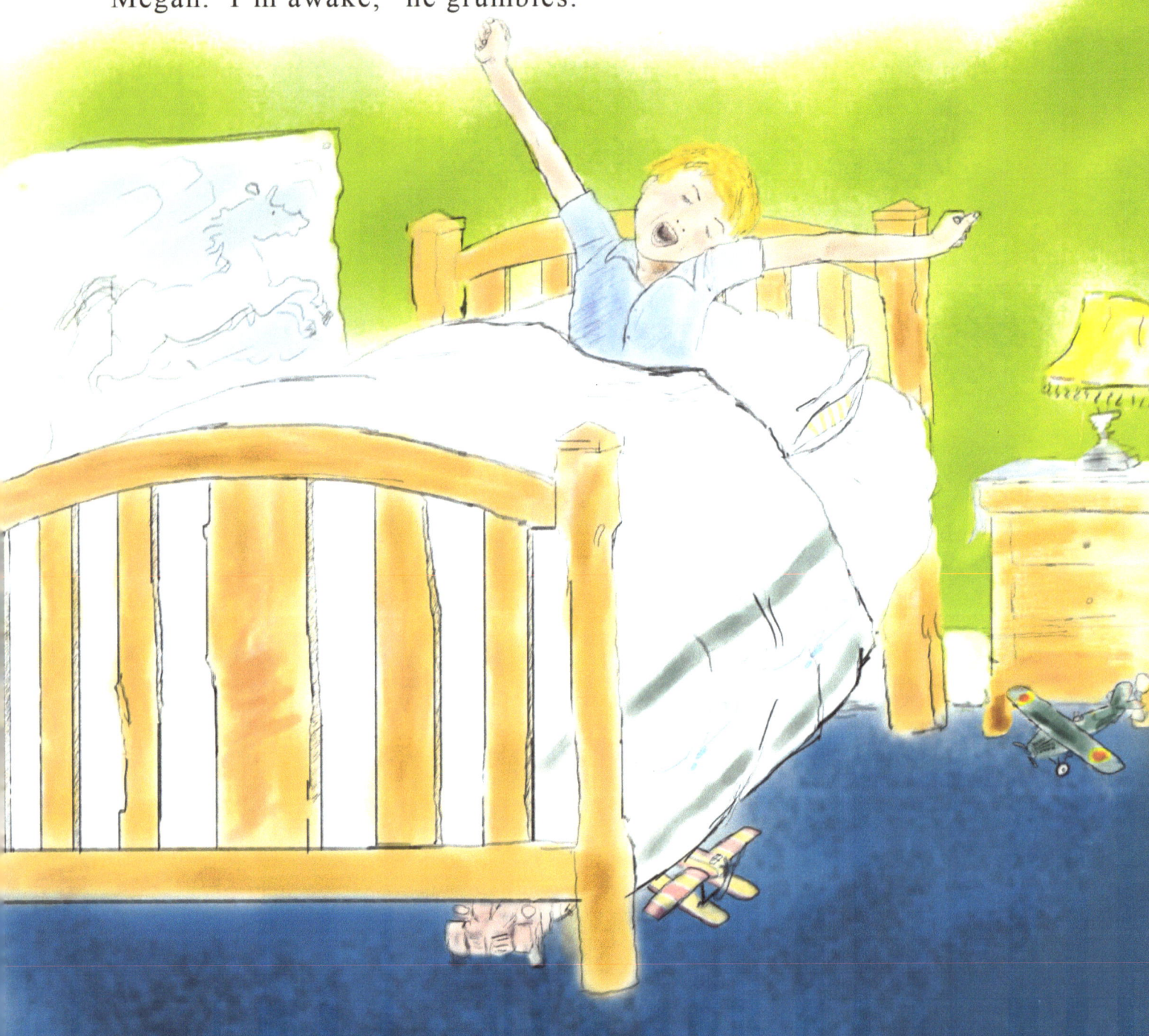

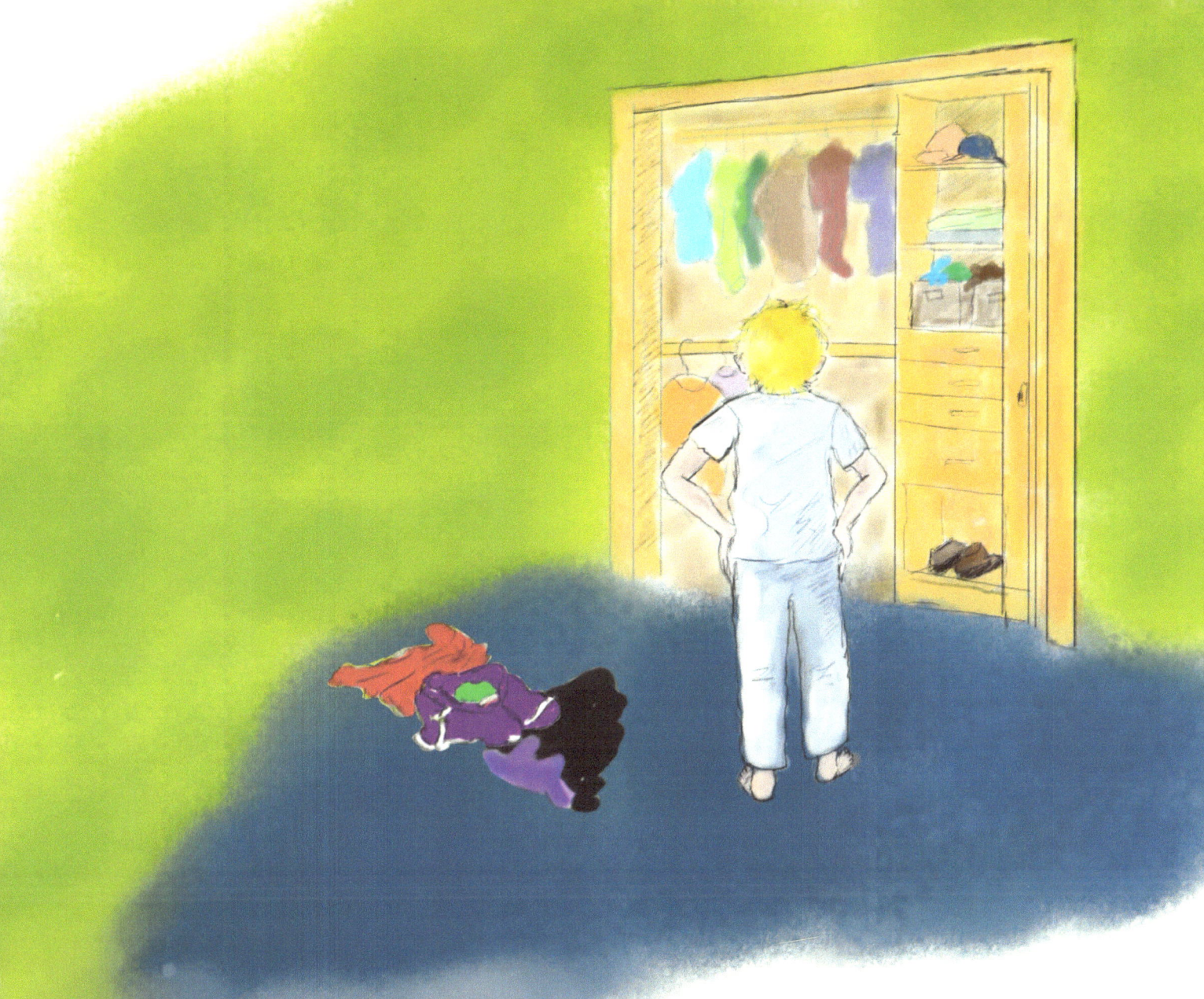

Jack needs to get ready fast. He gobbles down his cereal and ignores his sister's mean looks from across the table. As he runs back upstairs, his mom yells, "Don't forget to brush your teeth!" Jack hates brushing his teeth.

Back in his room, it's hard to decide what shirt to wear. The blue one? No. Maybe the black one? He sees his model airplanes and wishes he could play with them. "Jack! Come on," his sister yells. "I know! I'm coming Meg!" he yells back. He slips on his red T-shirt, grabs his backpack and runs downstairs.

On the way to school, Jack sits in the backseat while his mom and sister talk about something silly. Jack stares out the window. He is still upset about how Megan yelled at him that morning. "She doesn't get it," he thinks. "Megan doesn't understand that I have to do things my own way." You see, Jack is a little different. He has an extra Y. He has a condition called XYY.

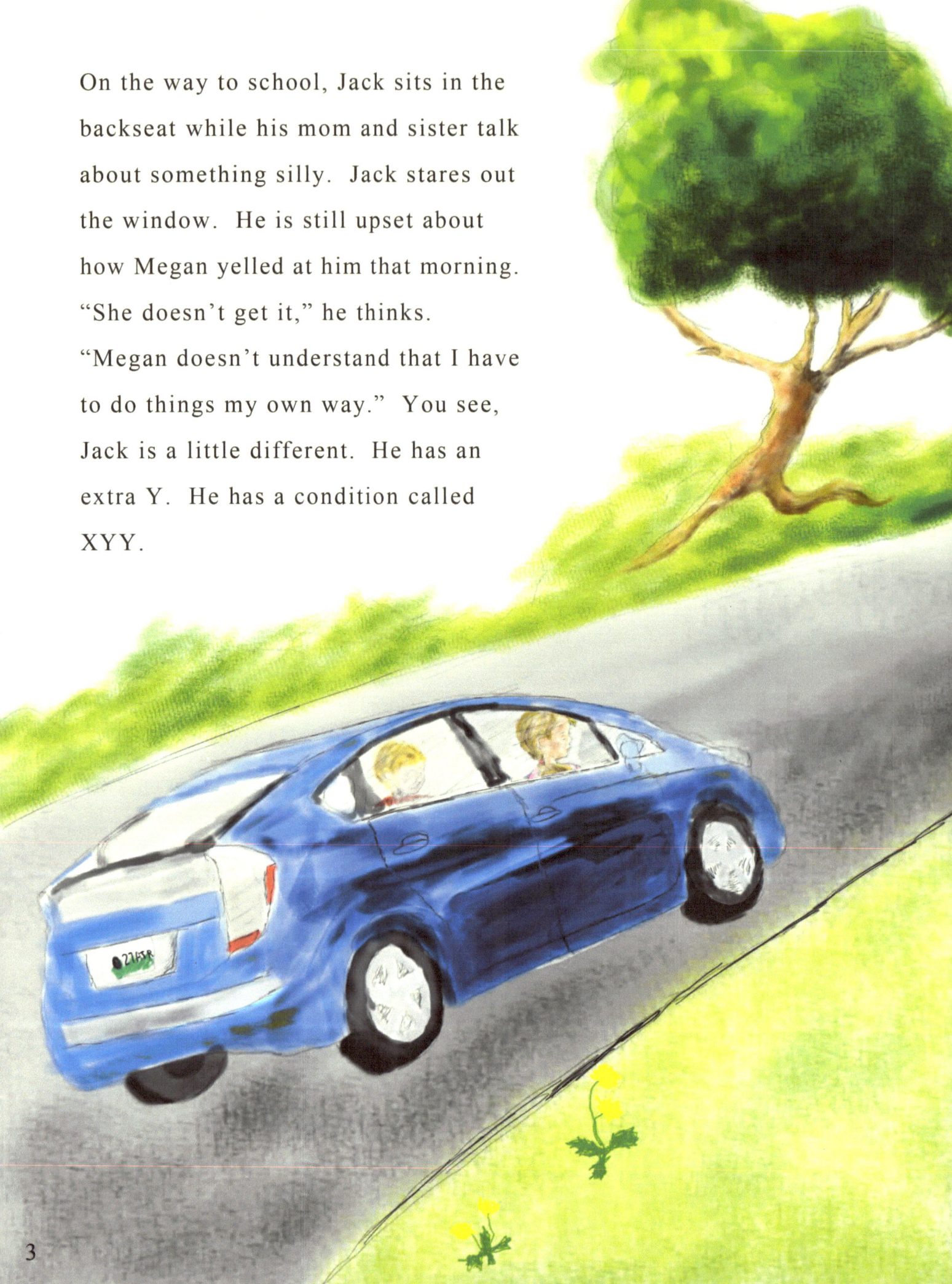

It all starts with genes. These genes are not the jeans you wear. These are the ones that run in families. Genes are in every cell of the body. They are the instructions that tell the body how to grow, what to look like and how to think and act. Genes are important and everyone has them, lots of them! Genes make people unique and different from one another. Without genes, people would be just faceless, brainless blobs of goo!

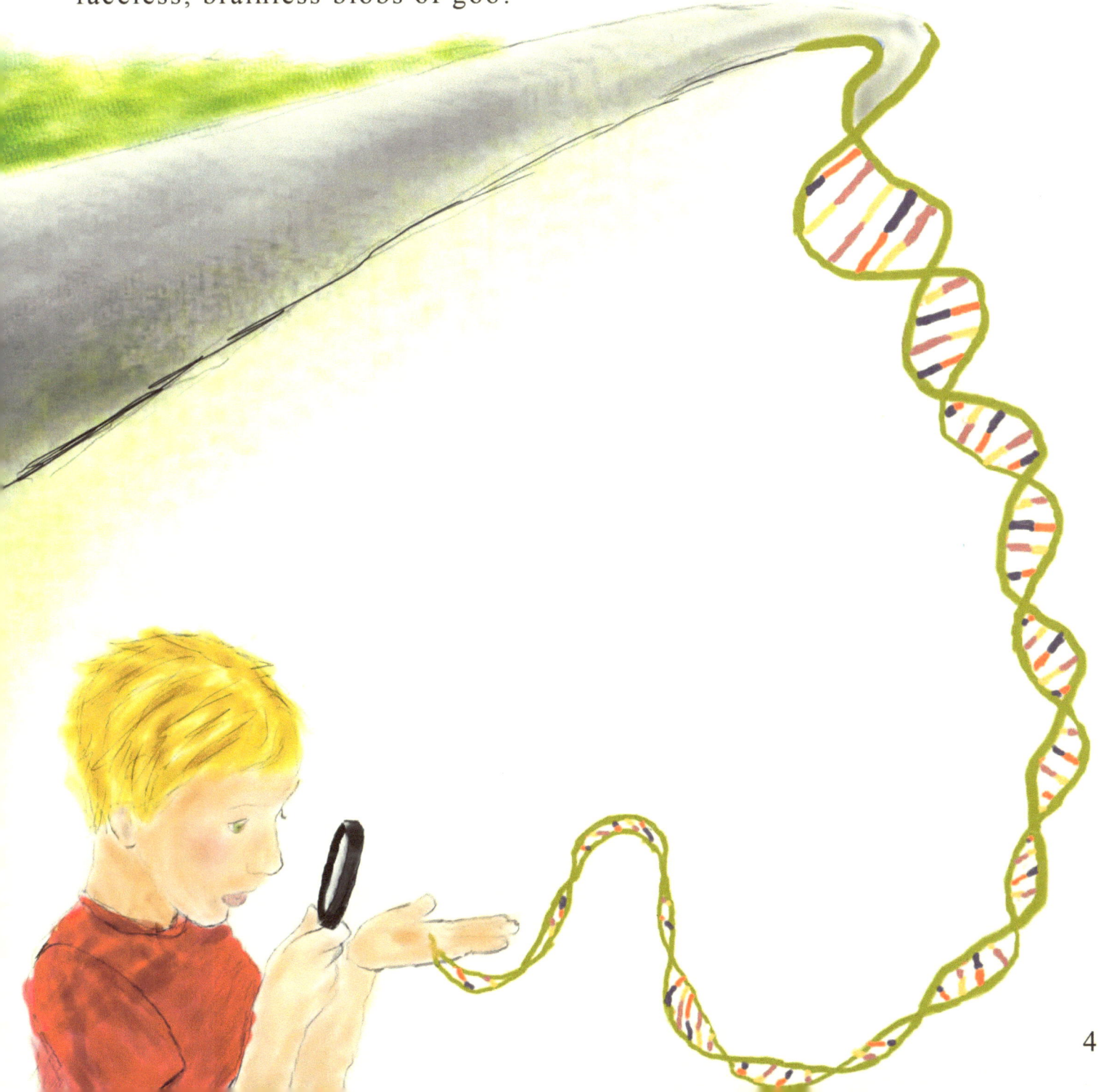

In the body, genes come in bundles called chromosomes. A chromosome holds a bundle of genes, just like a book holds a bundle of pages. There are too many genes to have just one chromosome, so people usually have 46 chromosomes to hold all of their genes. Chromosomes and genes are there from the beginning, when a baby is made. Half of the chromosomes come from your mom and the other half come from your dad. That's why kids look and act a little bit like both of their parents.

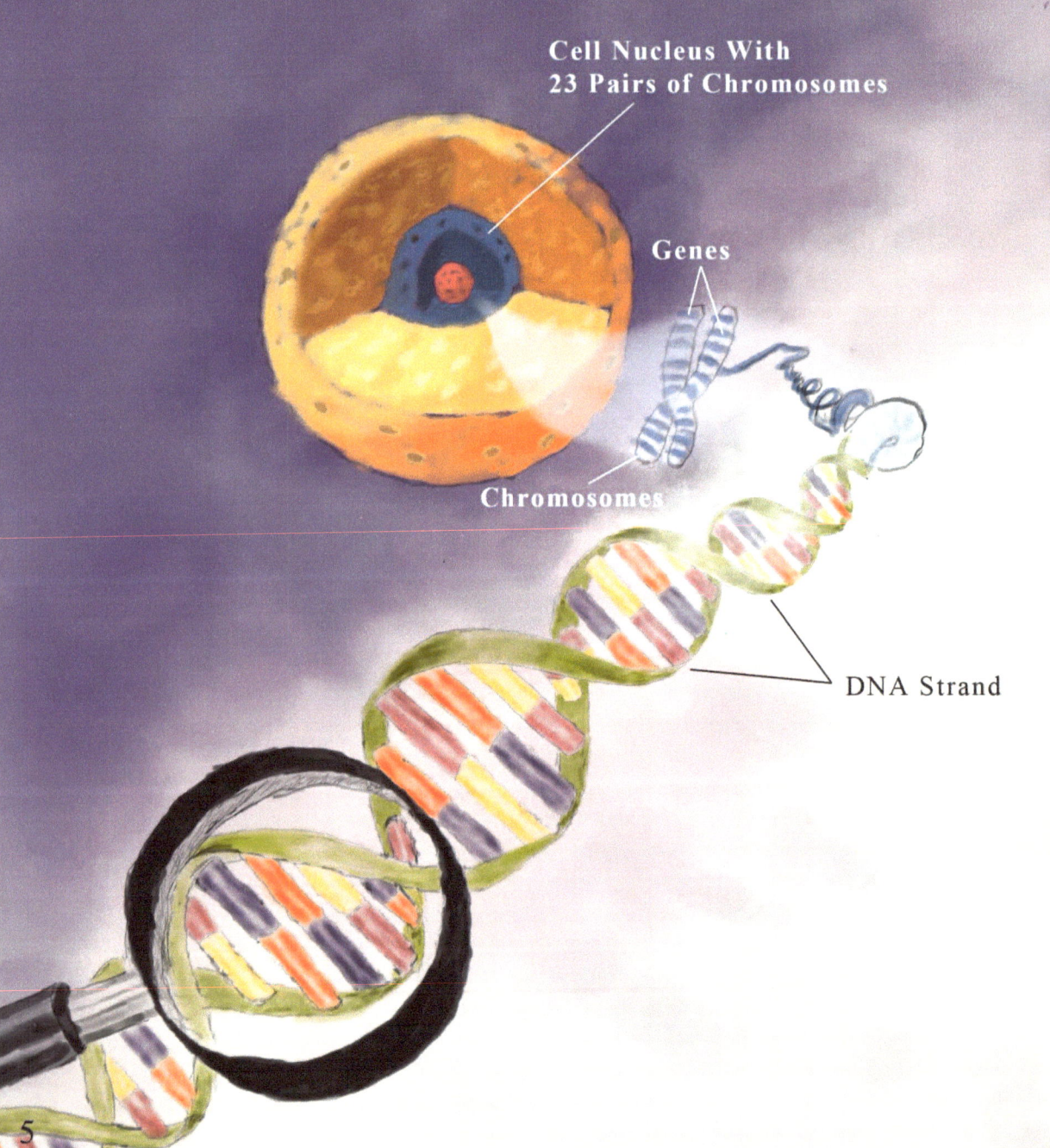

Cell Nucleus With
23 Pairs of Chromosomes

Genes

Chromosomes

DNA Strand

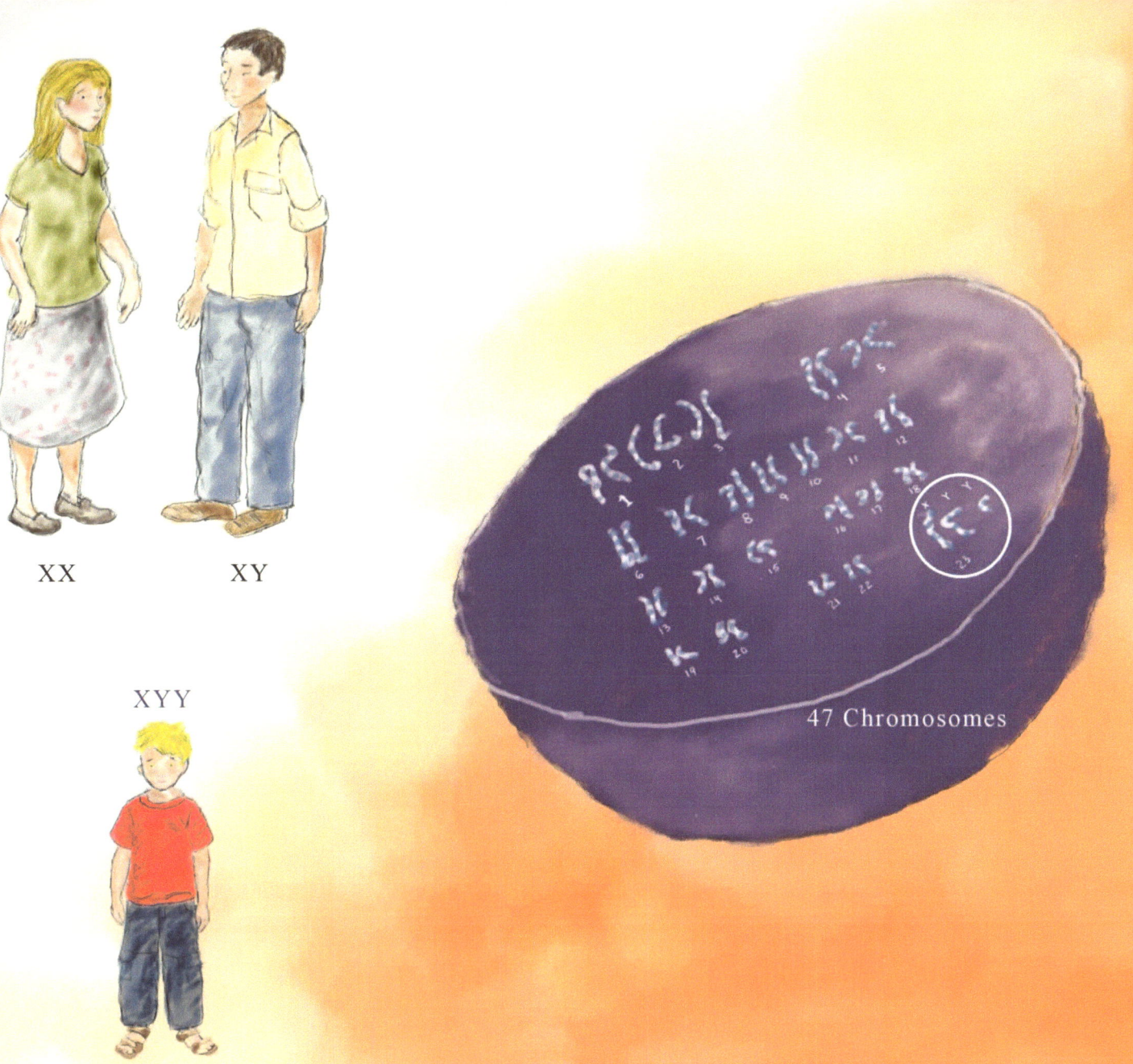

XX XY

XYY

47 Chromosomes

Usually, people have 46 chromosomes. Two chromosomes, the X and the Y, are different from the rest. It's these X and Y chromosomes that make boys and girls different. Girls have only X chromosomes, but boys have an X chromosome and a Y chromosome. It's that Y chromosome that makes boys look like boys. Jack is a boy who is a little different. He was born with an extra Y chromosome, his extra Y. So instead of having just one X and one Y like most boys, Jack has an X, a Y and an extra Y.

When a boy has an X and two Ys, like Jack, it's called XYY. Having an extra Y chromosome means Jack has extra genes in his body.

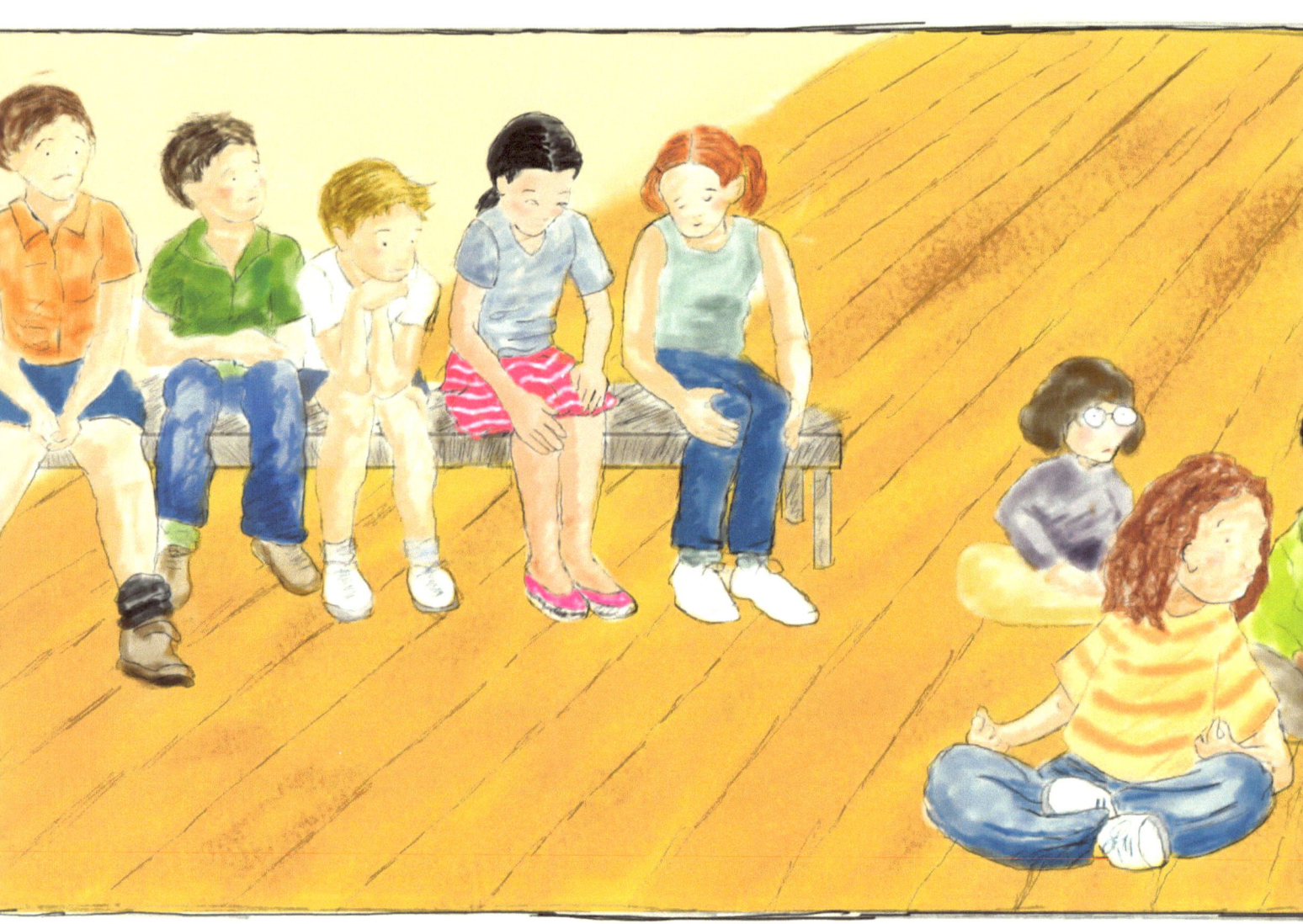

XYY isn't a sickness like a cold that you can catch from other people. Jack was just born with an extra chromosome. He isn't the only boy with XYY either. There are other boys with extra Ys. Some of them have the same challenges as Jack but some don't. He is not ashamed of his extra Y; that's just the way he is. Jack was made with blond hair, green eyes, smelly feet and an extra Y!

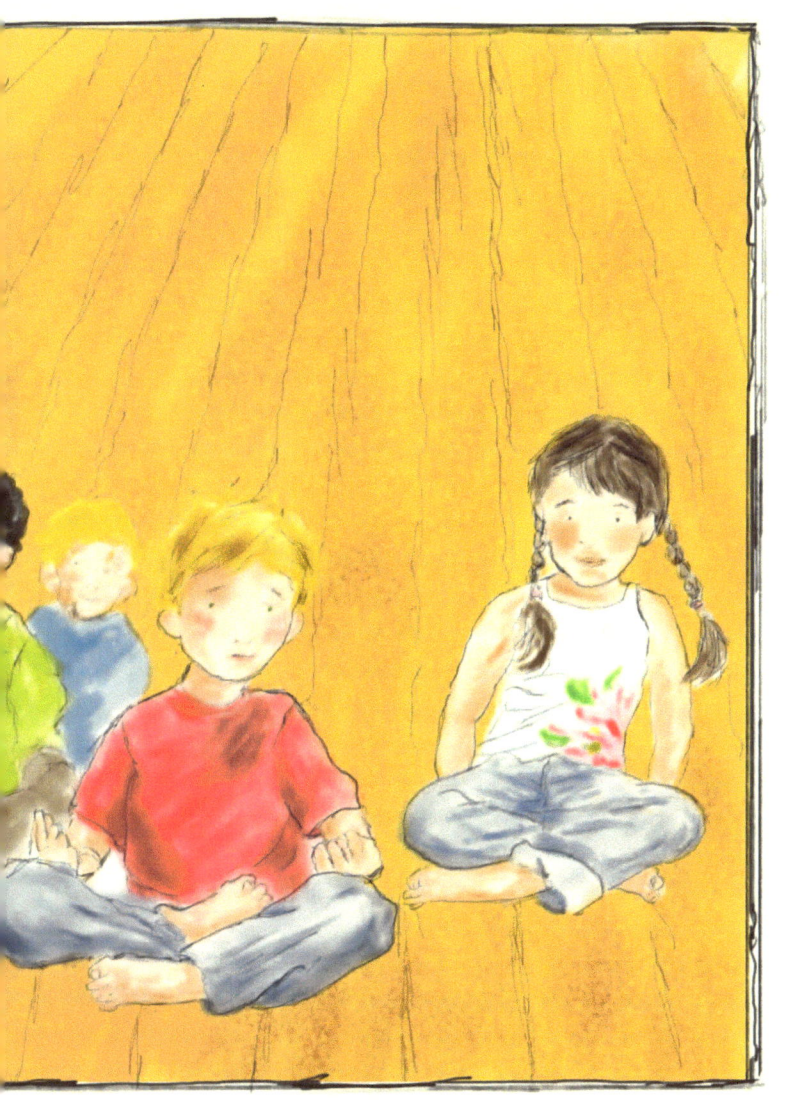

No one can tell he has an extra Y chromosome just by looking at him. He looks just like the other boys. But inside his brain, sometimes his extra Y chromosome makes him feel different. Sometimes having an extra Y can make things harder for him, like reading or doing school work. That's what Megan doesn't understand. She doesn't get that Jack is different. He has an extra Y and that means he has to do things a different way sometimes.

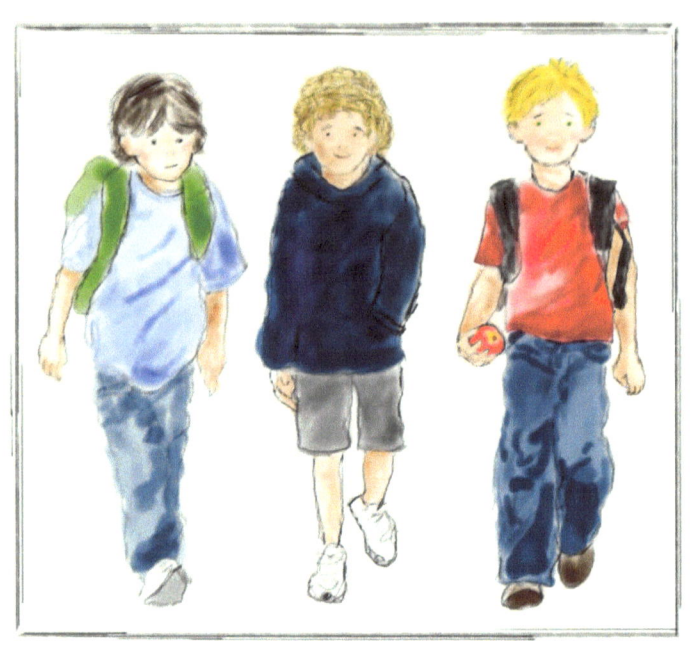

Jack's mom drives up to his school. He hops out of the car and sees other boys in his class. "Bye, Mom." He catches up with two boys, Sam and Johnny. They walk to class together and talk about their weekends. Sam went to the zoo with his family and saw a big giraffe. The boys talk and laugh together. Jack wants to tell Sam about the time he went to the zoo, but before he can put the words together, the boys are talking about something else. Oh well. Jack listens and laughs along with his friends.

The boys go to their classroom and find their seats. Jack sometimes needs extra help because it's harder for him to learn and remember things. His teacher gives the class 10 minutes to write a paragraph about their weekends. Jack gets frustrated and wiggles in his chair.

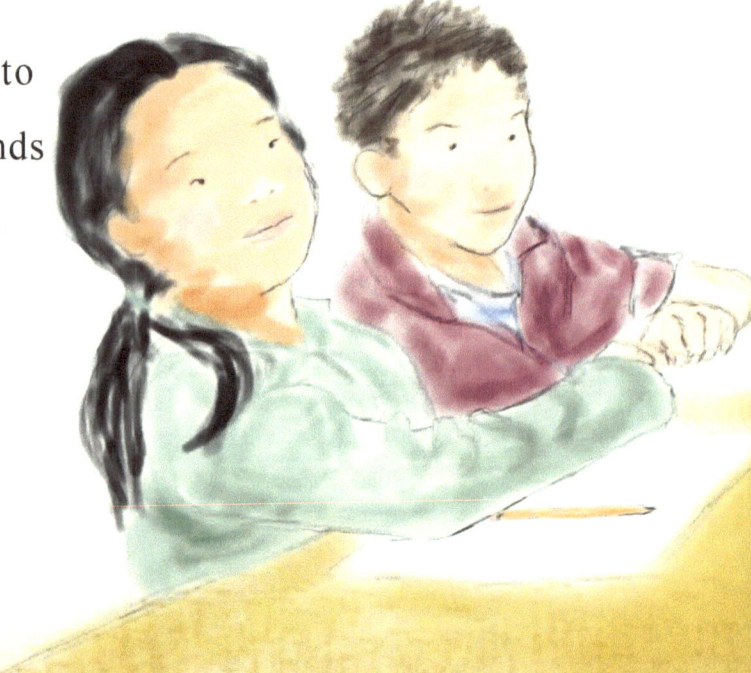

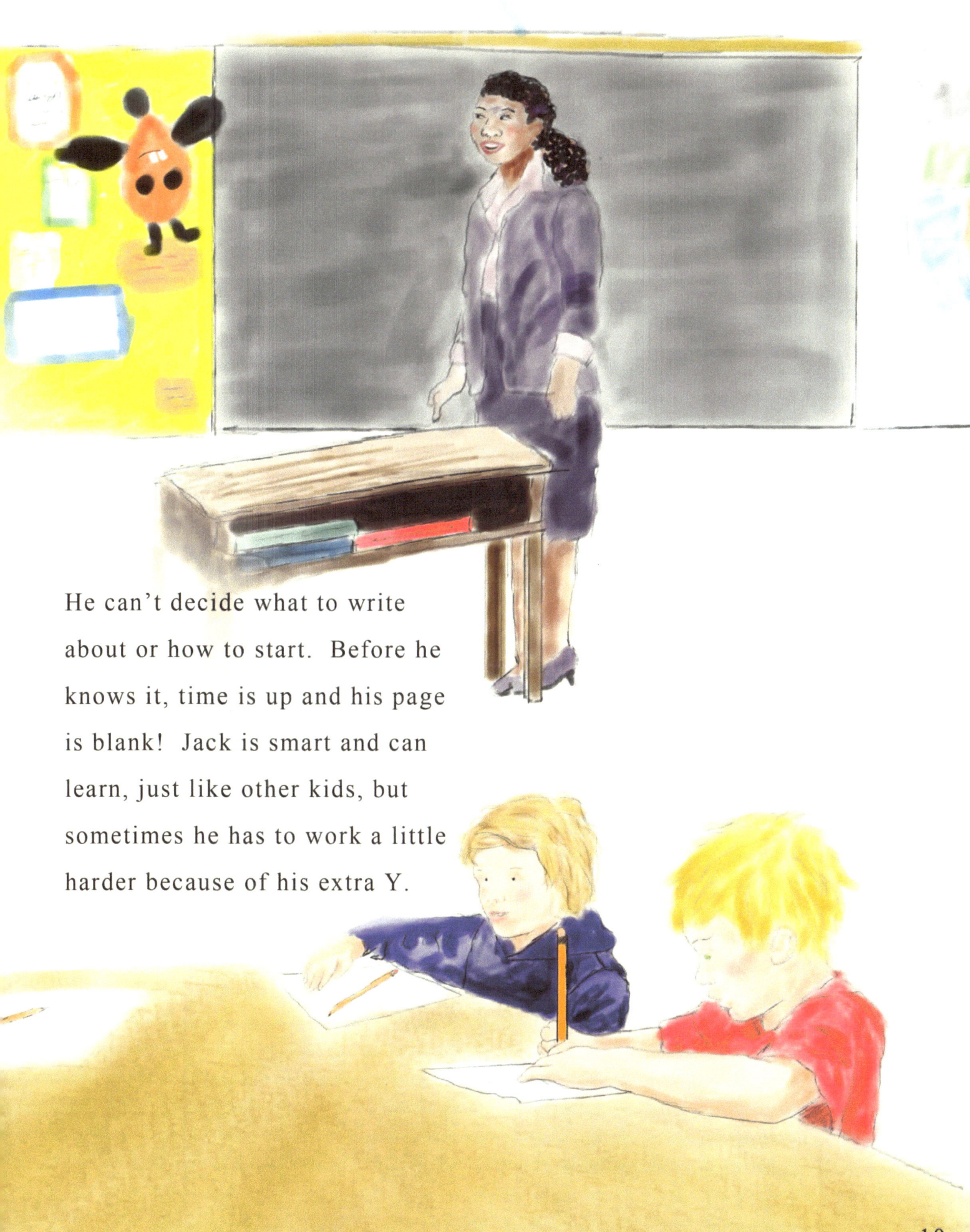

He can't decide what to write about or how to start. Before he knows it, time is up and his page is blank! Jack is smart and can learn, just like other kids, but sometimes he has to work a little harder because of his extra Y.

After lunch, Jack leaves his class to see his speech therapist. His speech therapist helps him learn to speak more easily. Sometimes people talk too fast and he can't keep up, or he blurts out things he's not supposed to say. Other times, it's like his words get caught in his brain, like when he wanted to talk about the zoo. In speech therapy Jack practices saying these words. The more he practices, the better he gets!

Jack meets with an occupational therapist at school too. Occupational therapy helps Jack practice using his hands to do things that are hard for him, like handwriting and buttoning. He likes to work on his drawings. Jack imagines all sorts of things to draw. He is the best artist in his whole class! And the more he practices, the better he gets!

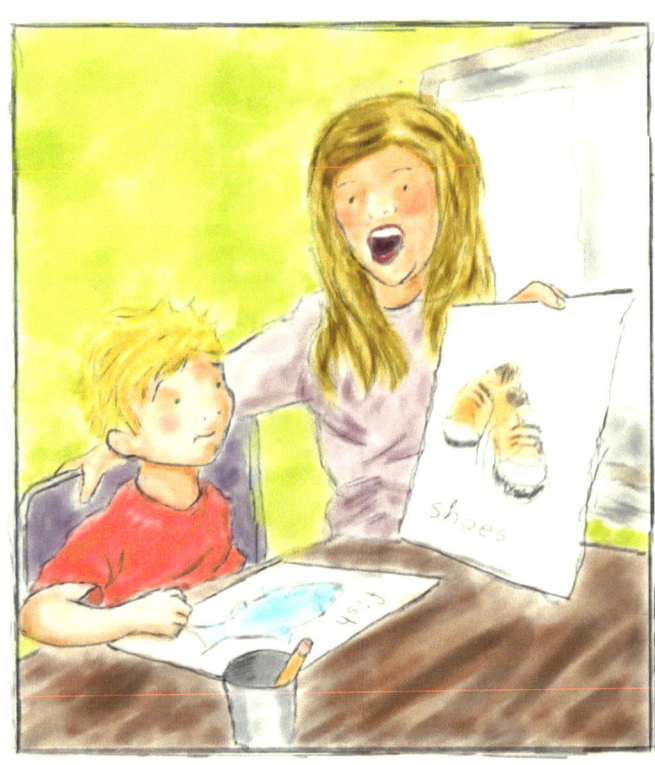
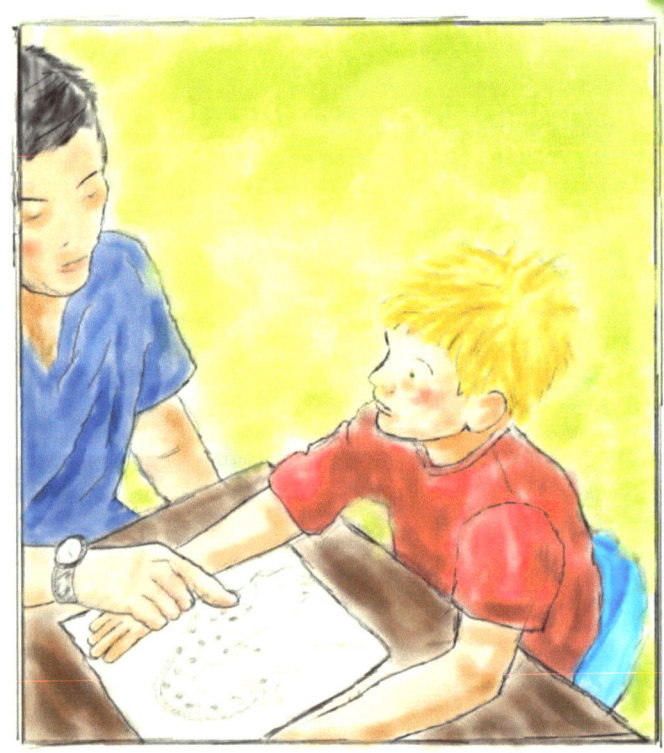

The school bell rings -- recess! He likes taking a break from class and being outside. He goes to the usual spot where he plays on the playground. Jack looks up and sees two boys playing tag, and they are running towards him! Nervous and breathing hard, Jack is glad when the boys swerve just before running into him. "Hey! Watch it!" Jack yells. It takes a while for Jack to calm down. He feels frustrated by the noise of everyone running around. He takes a moment to close his eyes and catch his breath. That's better.

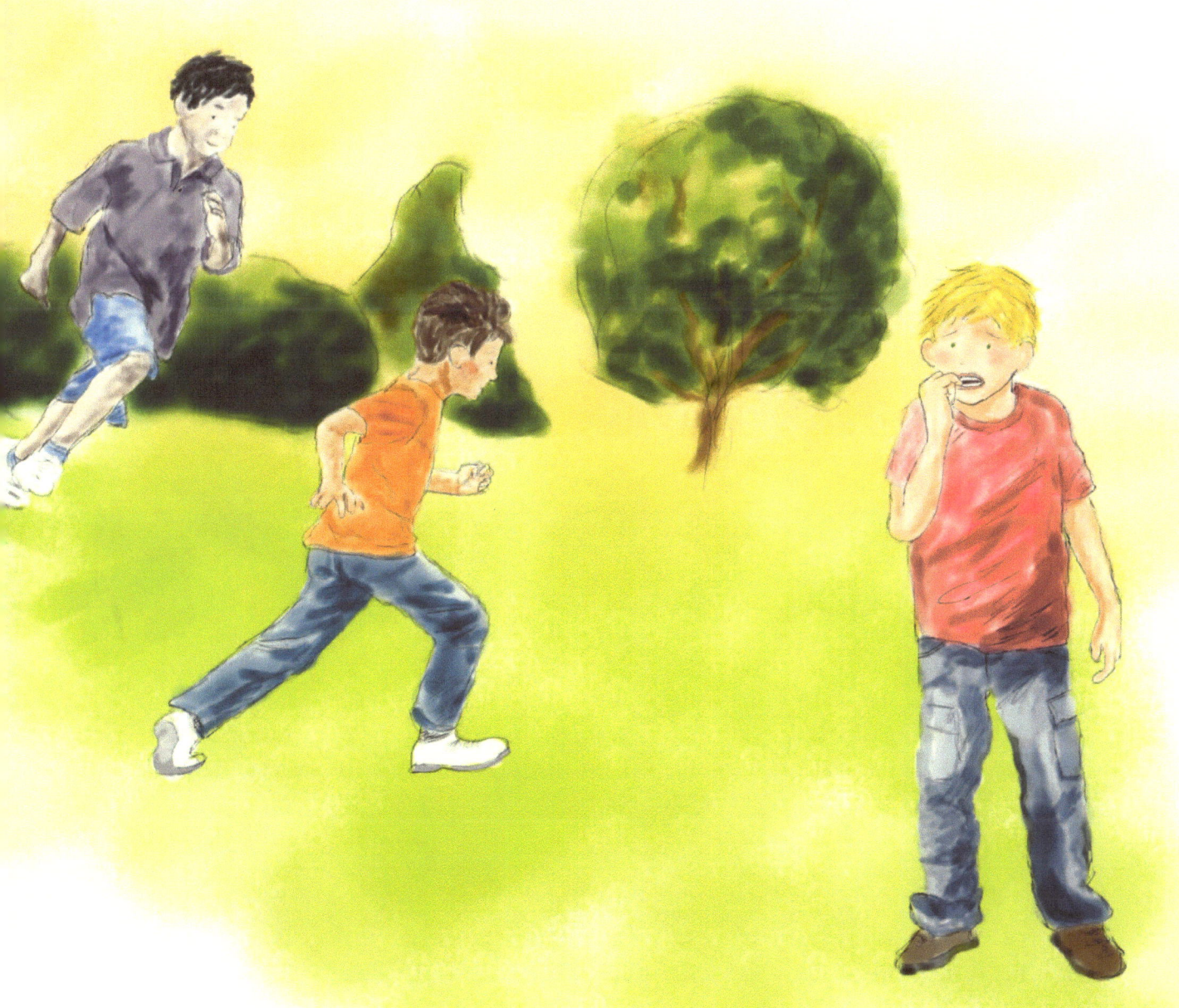

Ring! "Ah, man. Back to class, guys," his friend Sam says. The second part of the day is harder for Jack. His extra Y sometimes makes it difficult for him to concentrate. He takes medication to help him pay attention, but it's tough at the end of the day. Jack tries to listen to his teacher. It is easier to pay attention when they are taught interesting things or get to use the computer. Today his teacher is talking about something boring. He looks around and thinks about something else. The bell finally rings and Jack snaps back to reality.

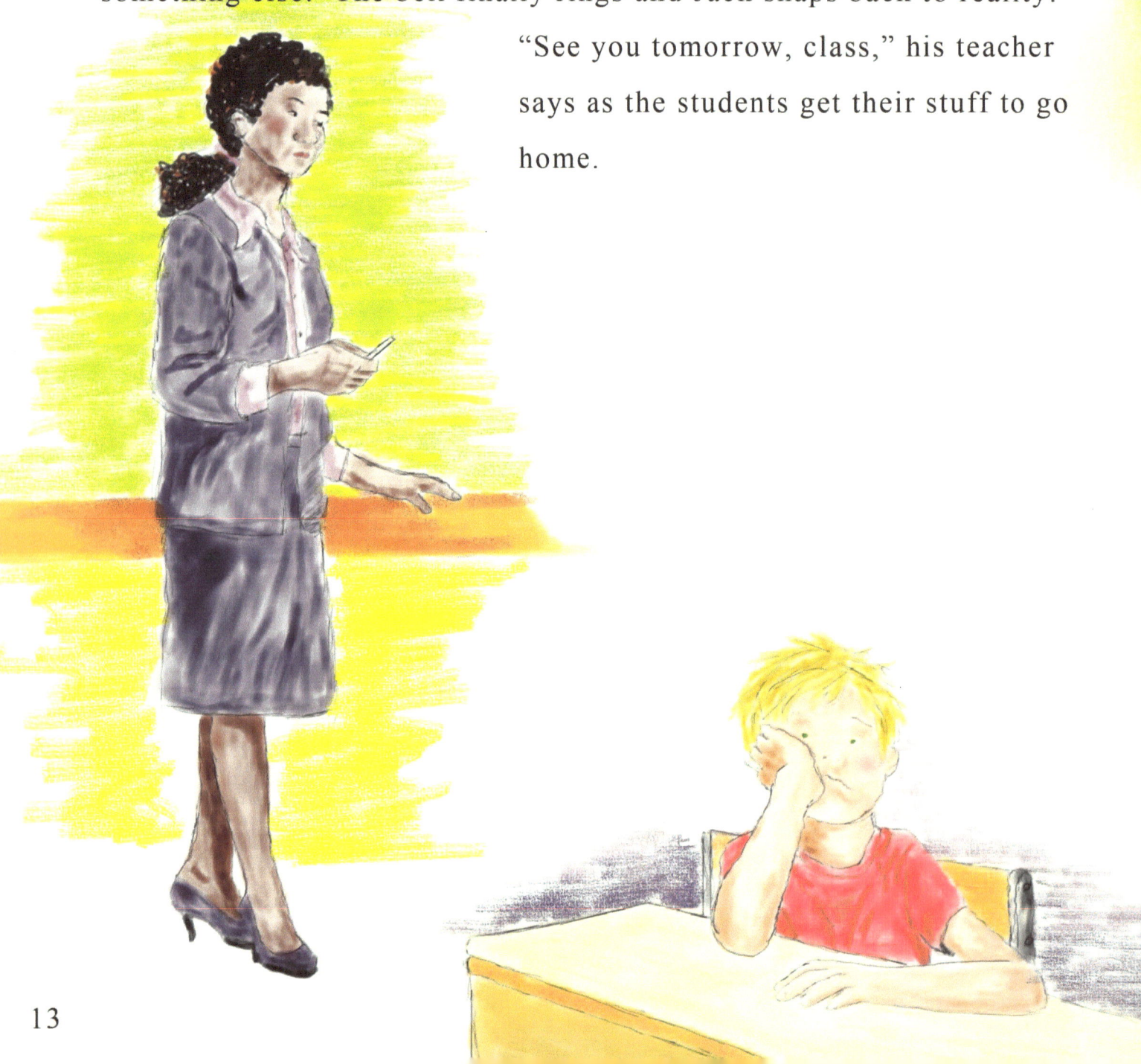

"See you tomorrow, class," his teacher says as the students get their stuff to go home.

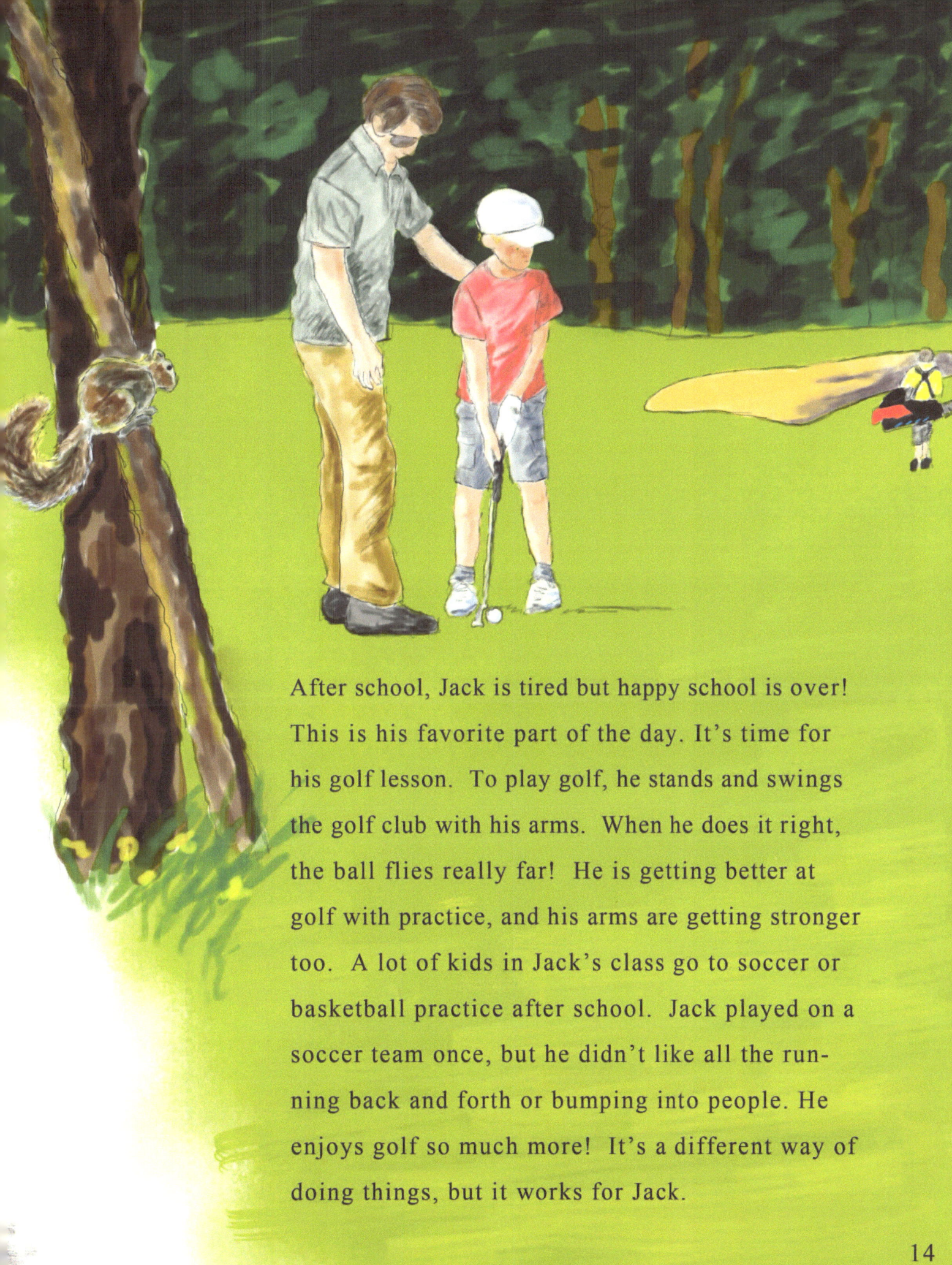

After school, Jack is tired but happy school is over!
This is his favorite part of the day. It's time for
his golf lesson. To play golf, he stands and swings
the golf club with his arms. When he does it right,
the ball flies really far! He is getting better at
golf with practice, and his arms are getting stronger
too. A lot of kids in Jack's class go to soccer or
basketball practice after school. Jack played on a
soccer team once, but he didn't like all the running back and forth or bumping into people. He
enjoys golf so much more! It's a different way of
doing things, but it works for Jack.

Tired from golf practice, Jack walks to the parking lot. His mom is picking him up to take him to his doctor's office. He sees her waving from her car. He smiles and waves back. "Hi, Mom," Jack says. She starts the car and says, "Hi, honey. How was your day?" Jack says, "Good." She asks him questions about his day, but he has trouble remembering the details. When he looks inside his backpack he finds the homework he forgot to turn in. "Uh-oh."

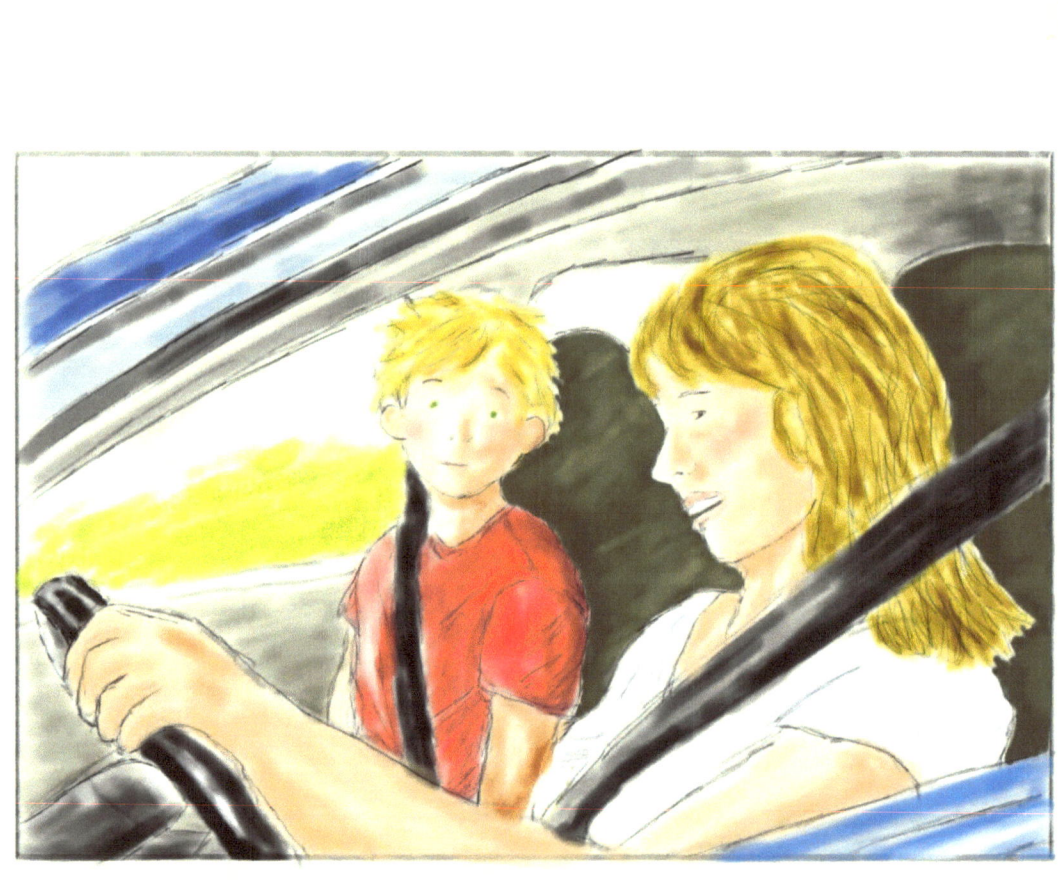

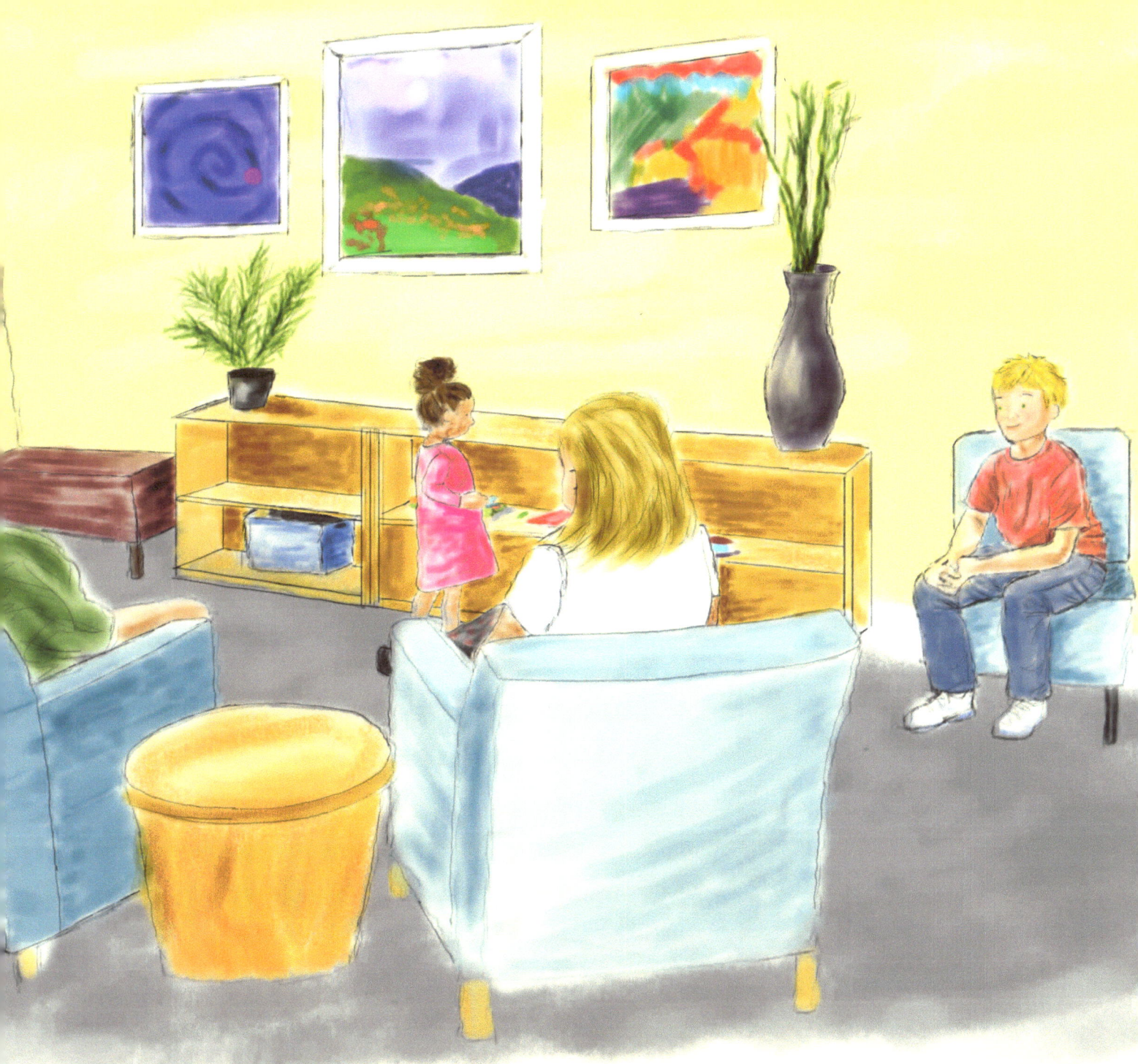

When Jack and his mom get to the doctor's office, they sit in the waiting room. Jack stares at the paintings on the wall. "These paintings are so ugly," he tells his mom with a laugh. "Jack, don't be rude," she says, but she laughs too. Jack has been in this waiting room many times before. Since Jack has an extra Y, he has to go to the doctor a little more than other kids. He doesn't go to the doctor because he is sick; he goes so the doctor can make sure he is healthy.

Finally, the nurse takes them back to the exam room. Jack sits on the doctor's table. The doctor comes in and has Jack lie down. She looks at his body, listens to his heart and looks into his ears. She pushes on his stomach which makes him laugh. "That tickles!" The doctor asks, "Jack, do you know why you have to come to the doctor?" He takes a second to think. "Because I have an extra Y?" "That's right, Jack. Boys with XYY can be tall and sometimes need extra help in school," the doctor explains.

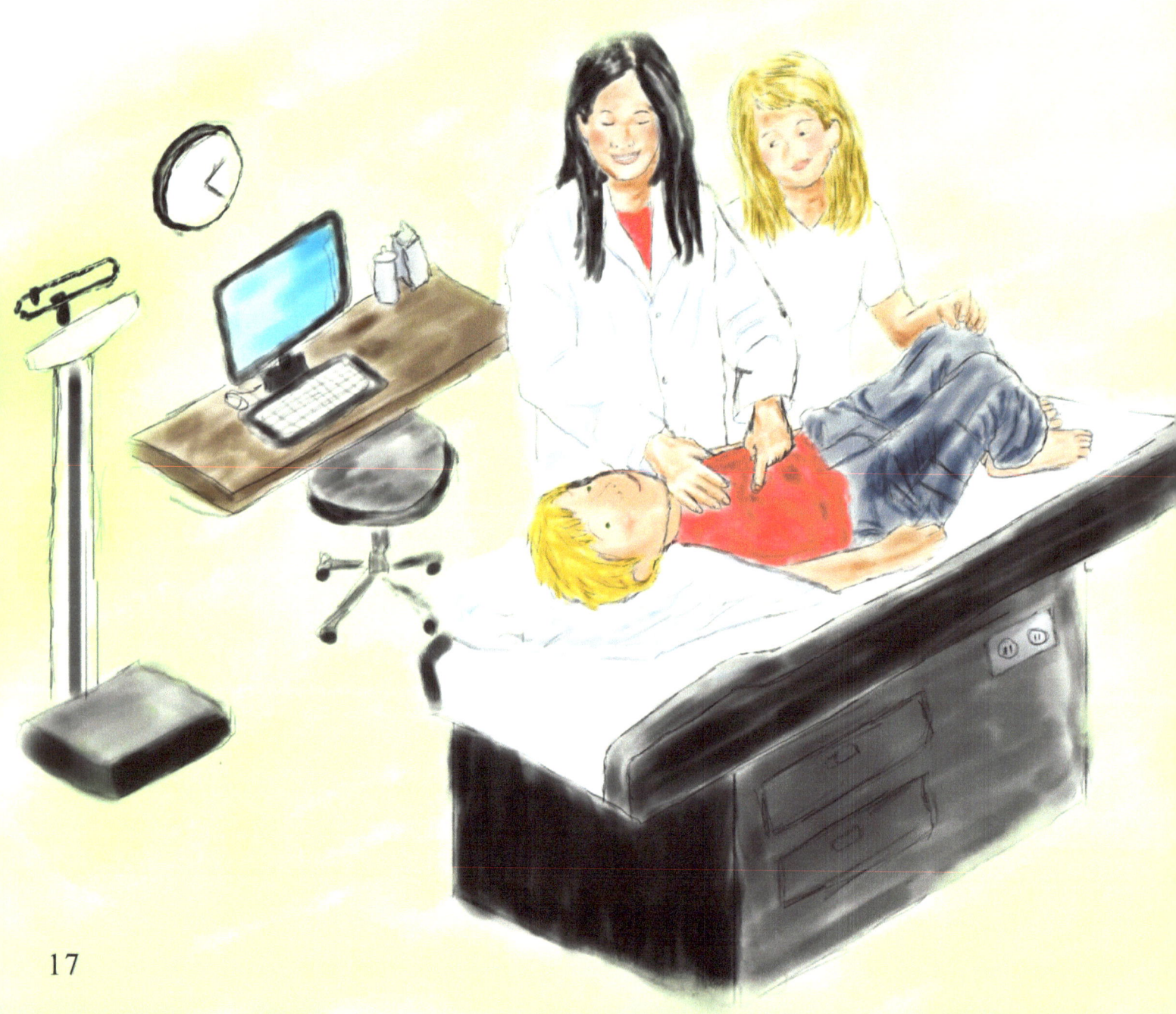

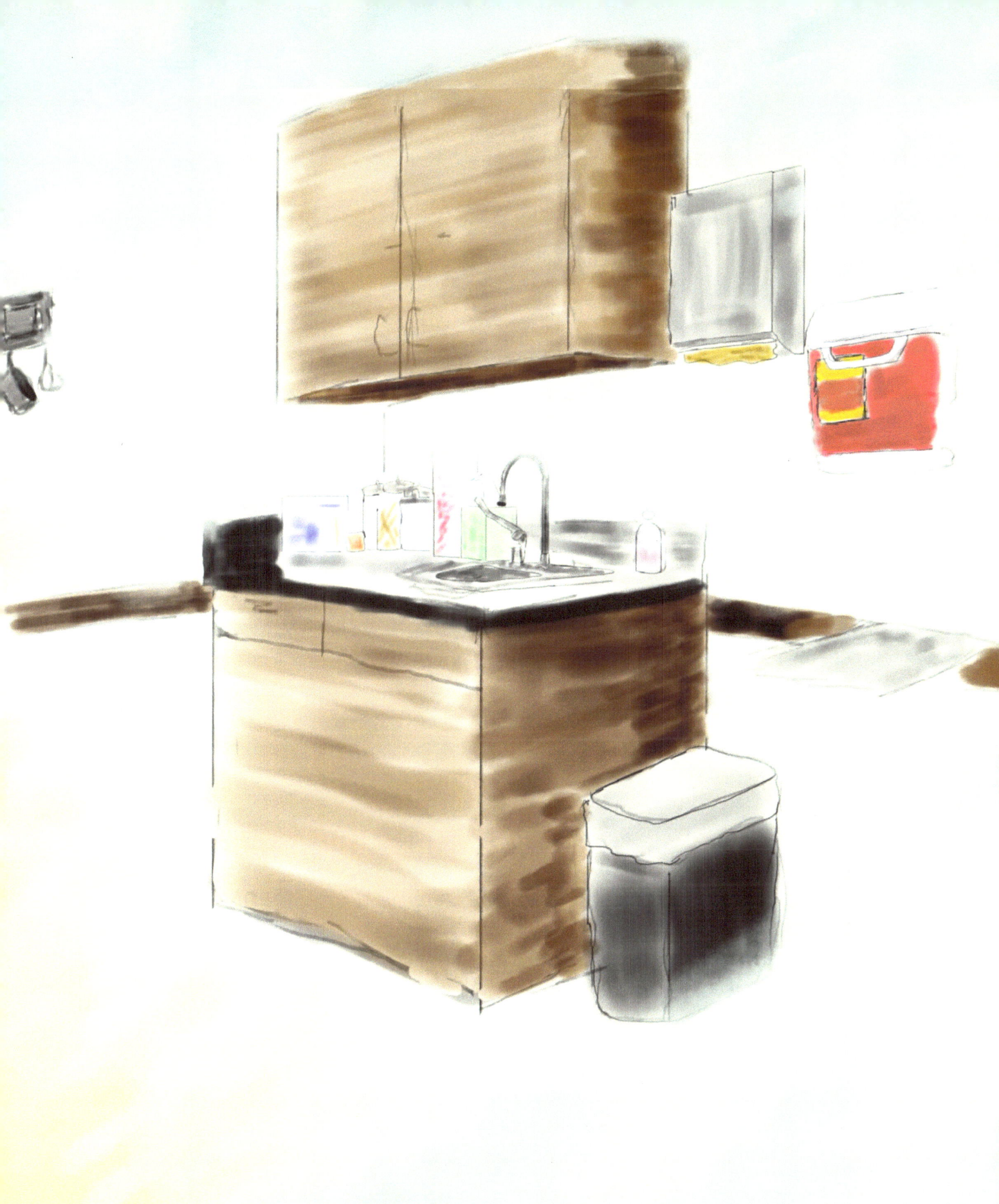

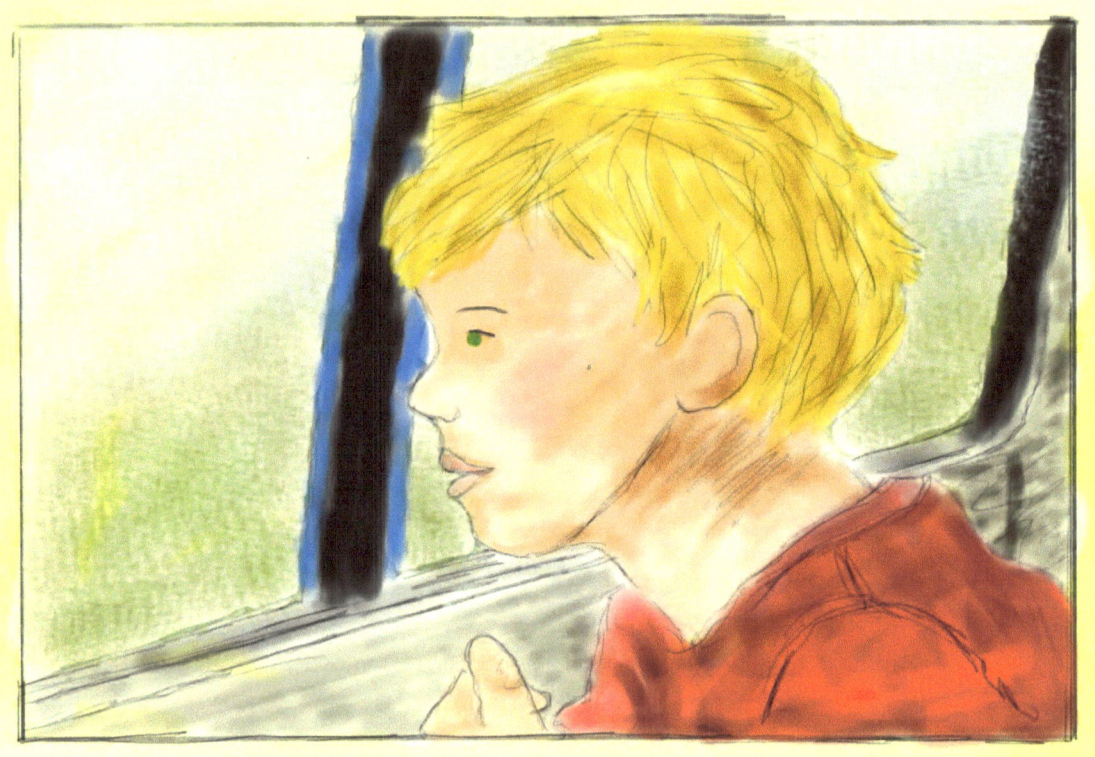

On the way home, Jack stares out the car window and thinks about the future. Jack is not sure what he wants to be when he grows up. There are so many things to choose from! He could be a farmer, or a teacher, or an inventor, or work on computers. He could be an astronaut and live on Mars!

Someday, Jack might want to be a father and have kids. Jack can be a father when he grows up, but because of his extra Y, he should talk to a doctor when he is ready to have his own kids. It's a different way of doing things, but it works for Jack.

Back at home, Jack and his family sit at the table for dinner. Megan blabs about her day. Jack is too tired to listen. He wants to finish eating so he can play on the computer. Jack's dad asks him about his day. He takes a second to think. "Um...well..." "Come on, Jack, I don't have all day," his sister says with a mean grin. Jack has had enough. Unable to control his emotions, Jack stands up from the table and yells, "Uhh! I can't stand you, Megan." Then he runs to his bedroom and slams his door.

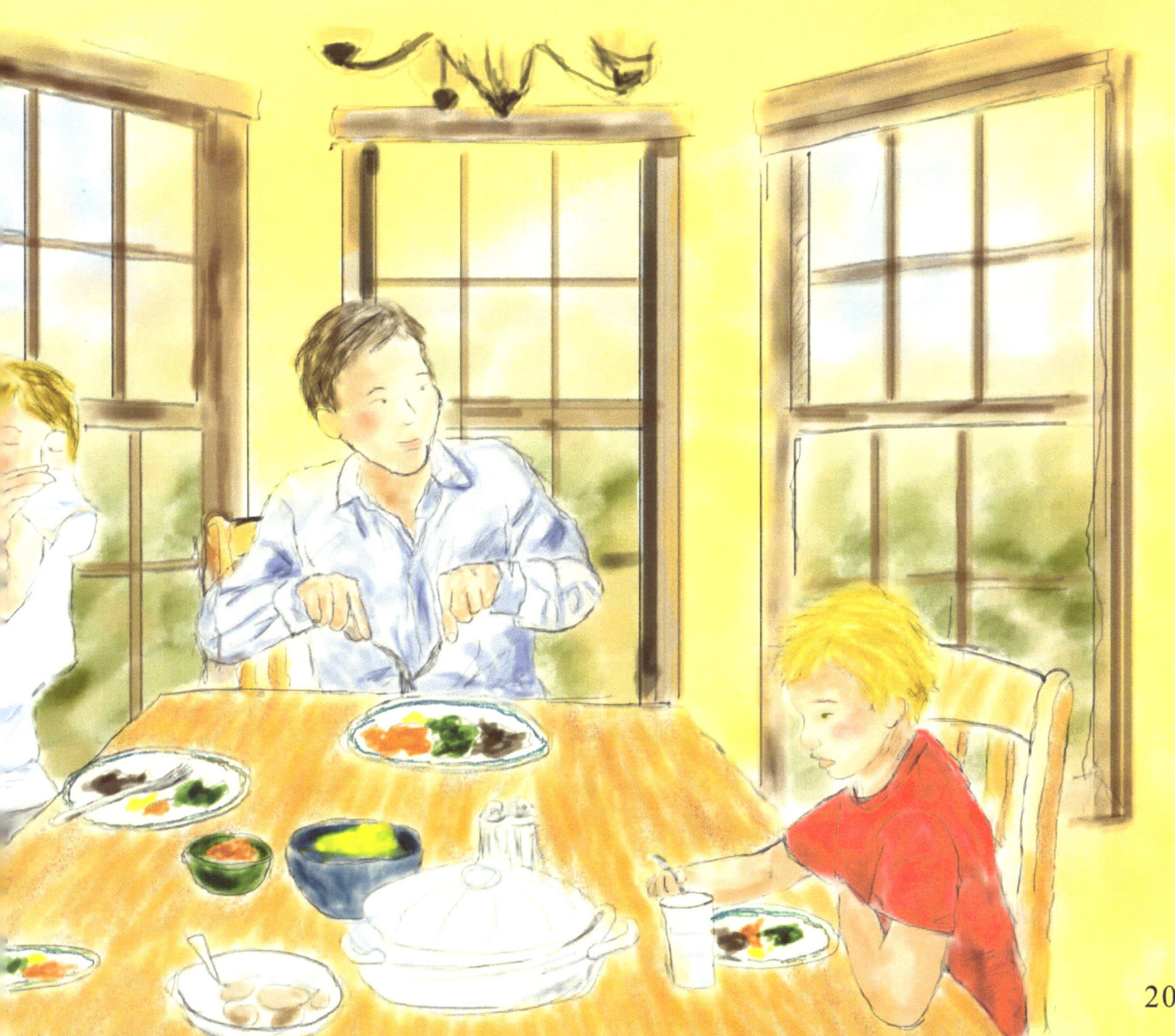

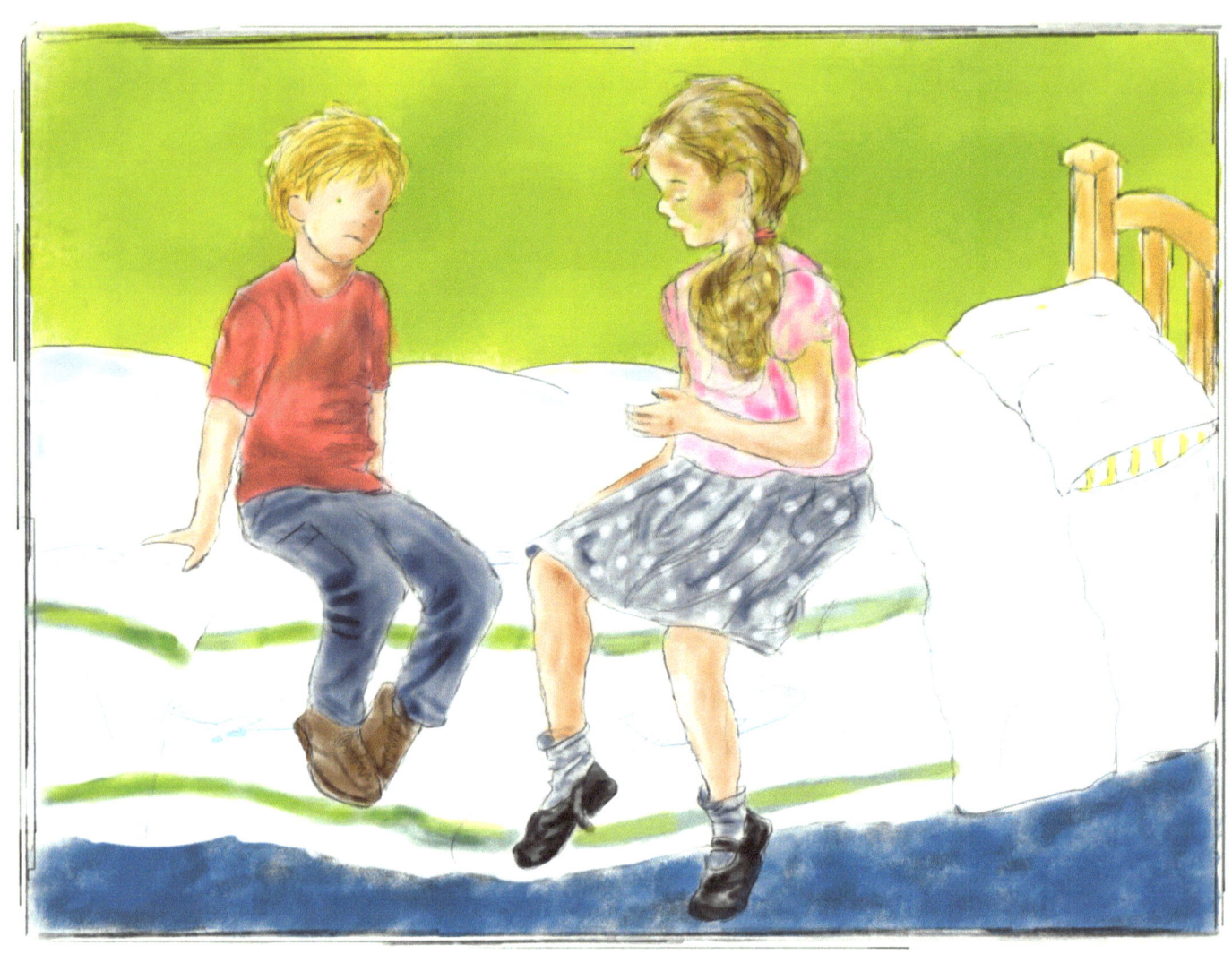

Jack feels mad and frustrated. "Why does she have to be so mean to me? Doesn't she understand that things aren't as easy for me as they are for her?" Just then, the door opens. It's Megan. "I came to say sorry," she says. "I didn't mean to make you so upset. I was just teasing." "Megan, you tease me too much. I'm different from you and I have to do things my own way." "I know. I'm sorry. It's important for you to be able to do things your own way," Megan says, "I'll try to be more patient with you. I love you, little brother." Jack smiles. "Yeah. I love you too, Meg."

It has been a long day. Jack's mom and dad tuck him into bed. They tell him they love him and close his bedrooom door. As he drifts off to sleep, he thinks about his extra Y. Having XYY is really just a small part of who Jack is. His extra Y makes him unique and different, just like all of his talents and traits make him unique and different. His extra Y is just one of many, many things that make Jack who he is. When he was made, he ended up with an extra Y. It's a different way of doing things, but it works for Jack.

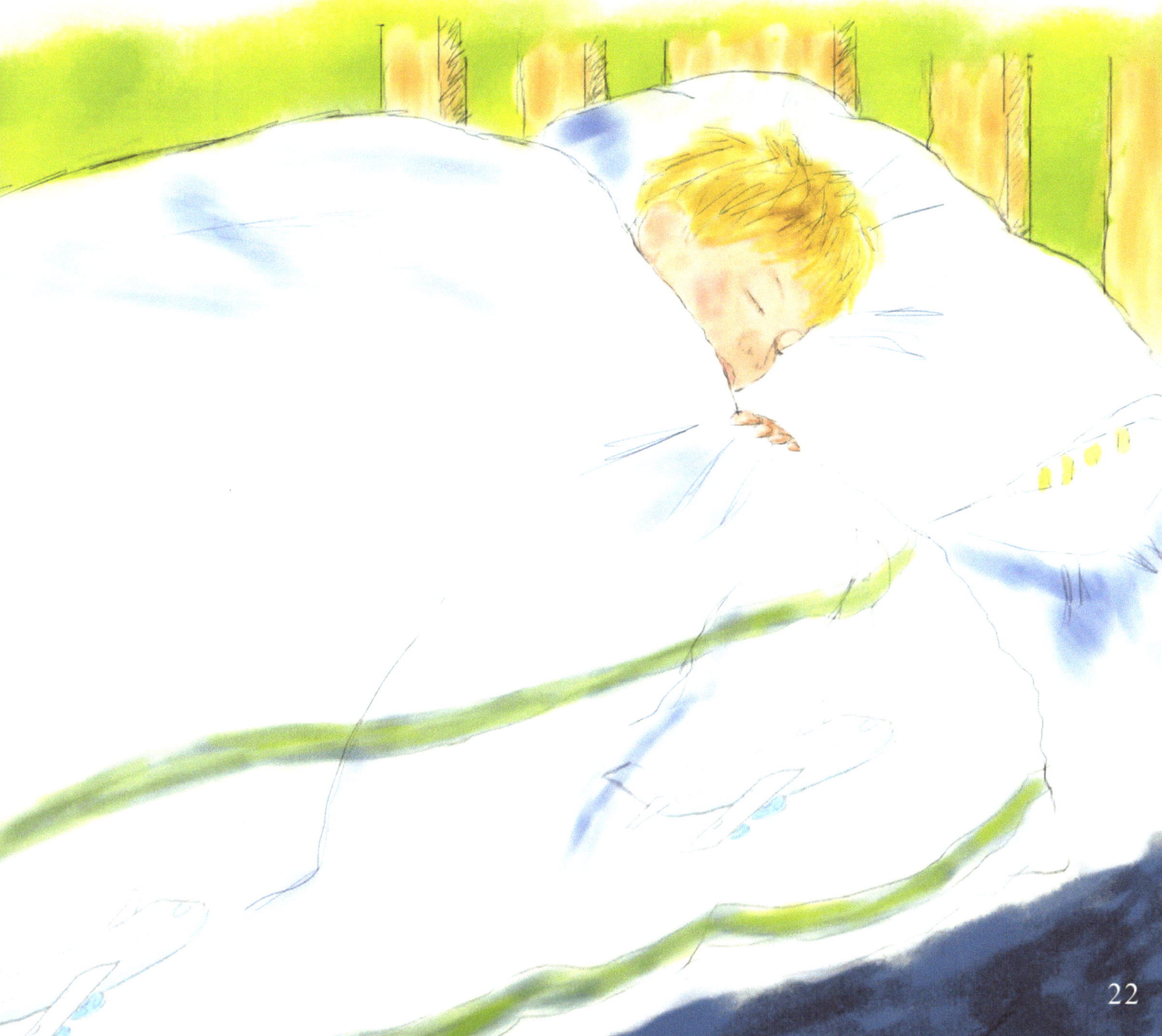

The end.

Acknowledgements

Creating this series of books would not have been possible without the time and dedication of many people who had a hand in bringing it to life.

Firstly, I am indebted to the many parents of children with X and Y chromosome variations who took the time to read the books between the time of their inception through to their final stages. The feedback they provided was so important in helping to craft the stories into ones that so many children will be able to relate to as they flip through these pages. Thank you for your time, wisdom and enthusiam.

I would also like to thank Susan Howell, Dr. Nicole Tartaglia and their colleagues at the eXtraordinarY kids Clinic, whose expertise and advice guided me through the creation of these books. Thank you for your patience, your encouragement and for reading these books almost as many times as I have.

Many thanks go to Suzanne Hayes, the illustrator of this series of books. With her creativity and talents, she was able to take my words and bring them to life in full color images. Her efforts turned my stories into children's books. I appreciate every minute of hard work she devoted to making this project a success.

My editor, Alexa McGuinness, deserves a great deal of thanks for remembering the grammar rules that I didn't and taking the time to read through every line of my books looking for them.

Finally, I would like to thank my family for supporting me in everything that I do and lending names to so many of my characters.

Arlie Colvin
Author

About the author

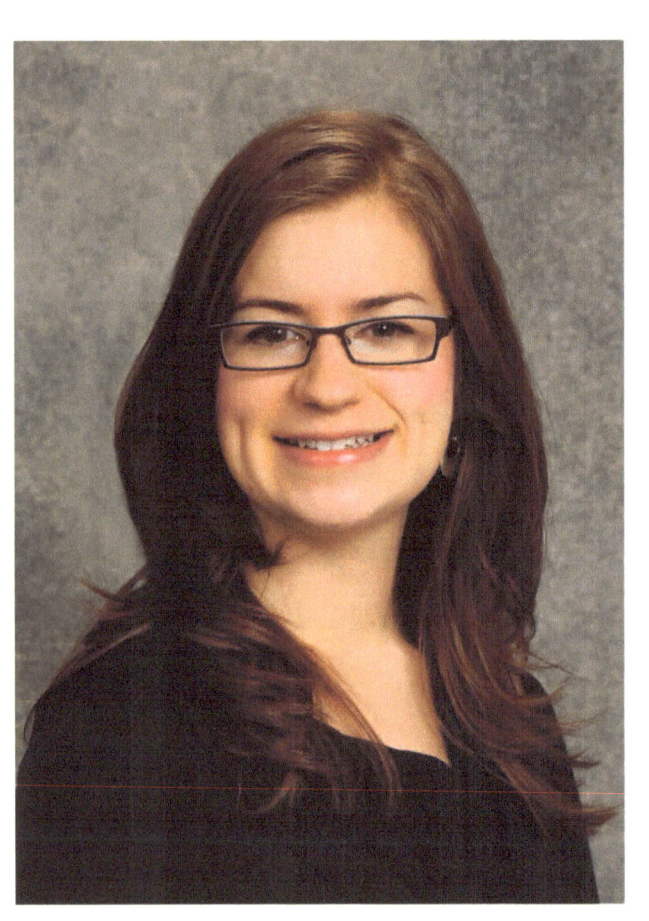

Born and raised in Muskegon, MI, Arlie
Colvin received her Bachelor of Science from
the University of Michigan. She attended the
University of Colorado Denver to pursue her
Master of Science in genetic counseling. She
became interested in writing children's books
for kids with X and Y chromosome variations
while working for the eXtraordinarY Kids
Clinic at Children's Hospital Colorado as a
graduate student. Arlie enjoys spending time
with her family, hiking and painting. She
hopes to have a long career as a genetic coun-
selor and children's book author, and impact
many people along the way.

About the illustrator

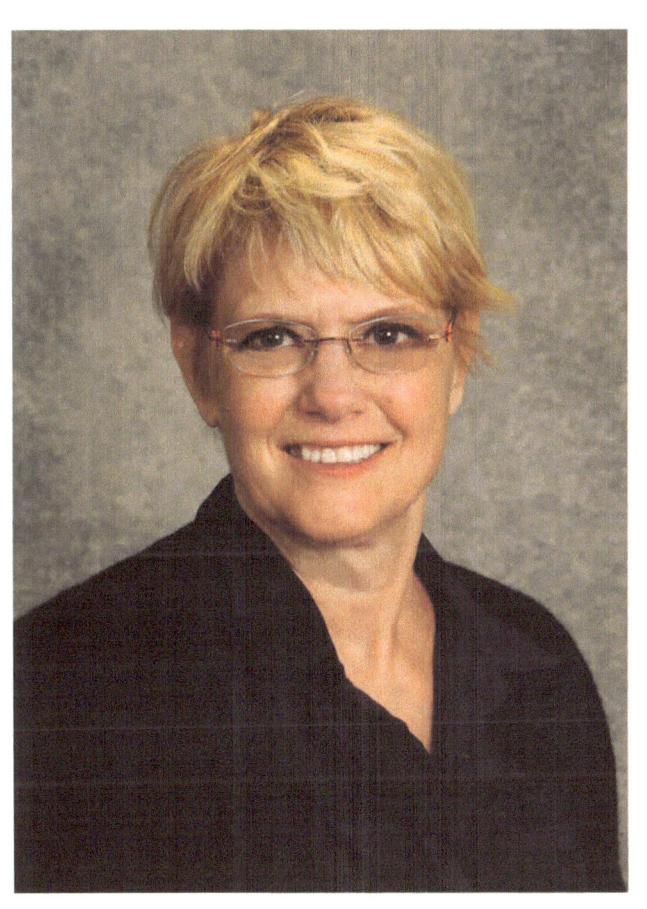

After a long career as an outdoor clothing designer and patternmaker, Suzanne Hayes returned to school at the University of Colorado Denver. She became interested in pursuing a Masters Degree in Medical Illustration in order to combine her artistic side with her love of the sciences. When she is not exploring the outdoors, she works hard at her art. She has especially enjoyed learning digital painting and drawing, using the storyline to come up with scenes that are illustative, corlorful and fun. Suzanne looks forward to having a long and successful career exploring the medical and biological sciences through illustration.